NATURAL BEAUTY FOR WOMEN:

BEAUTY AND ANTI-AGING SECRETS, ORGANIC AND INORGANIC SKIN CARE MANAGEMENT . HOW TO OVERCOME VARIOUS SKIN CONDITIONS AND HOW TO BE NATURALLY BEAUTIFUL WITHOUT MAKEUP

BY

ISABELLA NATHAN

Disclaimer

This book is designed to educate and to entertain. The contents are the sole opinion of the author. The author is not offering it as legal, accounting or other professional service advice. Although the author and publisher have made every effort to ensure that the information was correct upon publishing and at press time, the author and publisher do not assume and hereby disclaim any liability to any party, directly or indirectly, for any loss, damage or disruption caused by errors or omissions whether such errors or omissions result from negligence, accident or any other cause. The author or publisher will not be held liable for any physical, psychological, emotional, financial or commercial damages including but not limited to special, incidental, consequential or other damages. You should seek the services of professionals before making any decisions. You are responsible for your own actions, choices and results.

TABLE OF CONTENTS

INTRODUCTION   **PAGE**

INTRODUCTION

Take a look at anything related to "natural beauty"; the ads, magazines, websites, and billboards. They all seem to look a little monochrome. All the women seem to have the same skin tone (fair), the same shape (slim), the same hair (long, tousled). It is like there is one sole definition of beauty; one that leaves a whole lot of women out of the picture. Not to mention the fact that the beauty industry has gotten us all a little too focused on what is on the outside. It is all about fixing our perceived flaws (too wrinkly, too dark, too whatever) with products that they sell (how convenient). What about a more holistic view of natural beauty? One that cares just as much about our compassion as it does our concealer.

It is time for a new face of natural beauty; one that celebrates the vast diversity of people on the planet, encourages women to unabashedly own their style (whether that is a cat eye and red lip or just a smile), respects our values, and honors the fact that some days we just do not feel like putting in the effort (and that is okay). This book "NATURAL BEAUTY FOR WOMEN" embodies everything you need to know about natural beauty, how to identify various skin types, how to overcome various skin conditions (wrinkles, blemishes, cellulite, eczema and cellulite) and how to be naturally beautiful without makeup. It is a complete guide to natural beauty and a roadmap that leads you to achieving an astonishing look naturally.

CHAPTER ONE

HOW TO IDENTIFY DIFFERENT SKIN TYPES

It is vital to understand your skin type if you would like healthy and perfect skin. Knowing your skin sort permits you to pick out the correct product and customise a skin care programme that may work best for you. Your skin is your body's largest organ, as advanced and intelligent as your heart, lungs, liver and other vital organs. Using cleansers and coverings that are too harsh, even though they are suggested for excessive oiliness, may send the wrong signal to your skin that more oil is actually needed. Conversely, applying moisturizers which are too thick or heavy may end up in shrunken natural oil production, resulting in even drier skin. Taking the time to find out your skin's specific desires can assist you to decide on the correct choices that may balance the skin leading to a healthier, more radiant complexion. Every person's skin is exclusive, but there are a few common skin types that may help you to identify where your skin fits in the most. The 3 main skin sorts are ordinarily spoken as Oily, Normal/Combination and Dry. Here are two easy ways to determine your skin type at home:

The Bare-Faced Method

Cleanse your face totally with a gentle cleaner and gently pat dry. Leave skin clean (and do not apply any extra moisturizers, serums or treatments). After thirty minutes, examine your cheeks, chin, nose and forehead for any shine. After another half-hour, check whether or not your skin feels parched, especially if you smile or make any other facial expressions. If your skin feels tight, your skin is probably going dry. If there is noticeable shine on your nose and forehead, your skin is mostly likely normal/combination. If there is shine on your cheeks additionally to your forehead and nose, you presumably have oily skin.

The Blotting Sheet Method

This methodology is way quicker and sometimes a wonderful differentiator between oily and dry skin sorts. Gently pat a paper on the various areas of your face. Hold the sheet up to the sunshine to see what quantity of oil is visible. If the sheet picked up very little to no oil, you most likely have dry skin. If the blotting sheet reveals oil from the forehead and nose area, your skin is normal/combination. Finally, if the paper is saturated with oil, it is extremely likely that you have oily skin.

SKIN TYPES

Dry Skin

You may have:

- ➤ Almost invisible pores
- ➤ Dull, rough complexion
- ➤ Red patches
- ➤ Your skin is less elastic
- ➤ More visible lines

Dry skin possesses a tight feeling throughout the day, and may experience obvious flaking. Dry skin is basically because of patrimonial, environmental factors such as lifestyle & diet, hormonal changes, and climate. Dehydration is additionally a number one reason behind dry skin, so drinking plenty of water and avoiding diuretics like alcohol and caffeine can make a significant difference in how your skin feels and looks.

Daily exfoliation with mild, non-abrasive ingredients help promote skin cell turnover without removing skin's natural oils. Without an additional layer of dead skin, serums and treatments will be absorbed more easily. The best moisturizers for dry skin are those that contain hyaluronic acid (regularly listed as sodium hyaluronate in ingredients), glycerin, and marine actives like algae, because of their ability to attract water and deliver it on to skin cells. Emollients, together with squalane and bush oil, facilitate sleek and hydrate your skin equally and effectively.

Use these tips to help your dry skin:

- Take shorter showers and baths, no more than once daily.
- Use mild, gentle soaps or cleansers. Avoid deodorant soaps.
- Do not scrub while bathing or drying.
- Smooth on a rich moisturizer right after bathing. Ointments and creams may match higher than lotions for dry skin however are regularly messier. Reapply as needed throughout the day.
- Use a humidifier, and do not let indoor temperatures get too hot.
- Wear gloves when using cleaning agents, solvents, or household detergents.

Normal/Combination Skin

Not too oily and not too dry, normal skin possesses:

- ➤ None or few imperfections
- ➤ No severe sensitivity
- ➤ Barely visible pores
- ➤ A radiant complexion

Combination skin can have:

- ➤ Pores that appear larger than normal, due to the fact that they are more open
- ➤ Blackheads
- ➤ Shiny skin

Persons with normal/combination skin typically go through xerotes on the cheeks, making it more vital to find a moisturizer that is not too heavy but one substantial enough to retain moisture where needed most. Those with traditional skin are not at risk of breakouts on their cheeks, and tend to have a well-moisturized t-zone. Gentle, daily exfoliation is additionally necessary to make the t-zone and cheek areas balance. Moisturizers with a gel-like texture are been absorbed a lot quicker and not likely to cause breakouts. Start with a little quantity and increase gradually to the required level to avoid over-moisturizing and stressing the skin.

Oily Skin

You may have:

> ➤ Enlarged pores
>
> ➤ Dull or shiny, thick complexion
>
> ➤ Blackheads, pimples, or other blemishes

Oiliness can vary depending upon the time of year or the weather. Things that can cause or worsen it include:

> ➤ Puberty or other hormonal imbalances
>
> ➤ Stress
>
> ➤ Heat or too much humidity

To take care of oily skin:

> ➤ It should be washed not more than 2 times a day and after you sweat a lot.
>
> ➤ Use a gentle cleanser and do not scrub.
>
> ➤ Do not pick, pop, or squeeze pimples. They will take longer to heal.
>
> ➤ Find the word "noncomedogenic" on skin care products and cosmetics. This entails it will not clog pores.

Excess oil will often leave pores full and clogged. One good thing is that oily skin appears younger and much more supple because it possesses a lot of natural wetness and it is less prone to wrinkles. Daily enzymatic exfoliation is important to encourage cell turnover and stop secretion buildup in pores. A gentle physical exfoliator (that does not use abrasives like crushed nuts or seeds that may cause little tears within the dermis) is additionally helpful for equalization of the tone and texture of your skin.

Oilier skin is also prone to PIH (post-inflammatory hyper pigmentation), a condition which leaves dark spots on the skin after a breakout has healed. Exfoliation will also help lighten these dark spots by polishing away the uppermost layers of skin and revealing new cells. Those with moderate to severe acneic breakouts ought to think about employing an exfoliator that contains anti-bacterial ingredients to quicken healing and stop future blemishes.

HOW TO OVERCOME WRINKLES

Creases (wrinkles) are not good to look, be it on your clothes or on your face! The beginning of wrinkles, probably the one thing no one ever wishes to experience. Smooth skin will be a proof of health, vitality, and youth. Many people strive through other ways to make their skin wrinkle-free as they age. Wrinkles will develop on your skin because of age, exposure to ultraviolet light, smoking, and repeated facial gestures such as smiling or squinting. Although there exist several anti-wrinkle creams, serums, and supplements available, you may prefer natural ways to get rid of your wrinkles. You can do that by keeping your skin wet, encouraging firmer skin with lifestyle choices, and preventing wrinkles from forming in the first place.

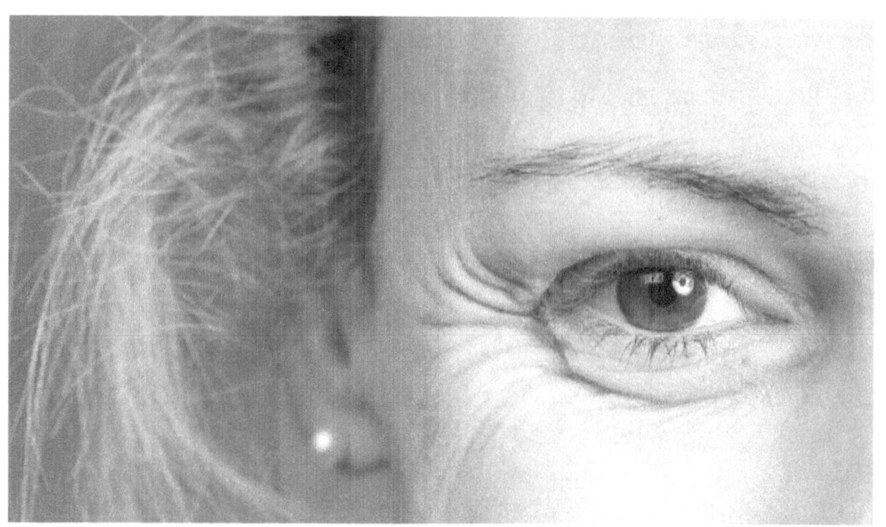

What Are Wrinkles?

Wrinkles are also known as rhytides. They are creases within the skin that become pronounced with aging because the skin loses its natural physical property.

Signs & Symptoms

> Fine lines close to the eyes, mouth, and around the neck

> Skin sags in distinct areas, especially on the face and neck

> The skin on the hands are loose

> Deep wrinkles around the eyes and lips

What Causes Wrinkles on Skin?

As you age, your skin tends to lose its physical property and wetness. These wrinkles typically appear perpendicular to the underlying muscles. For example, frown lines of the forehead are horizontal, and the underlying frontalis muscle is a vertically oriented muscle. The elastin and collagen fibers start to degrade, and as we age, we lose our ability to repair the collagen fibers. The lack of those 2 factors is the prime reason for the birth of wrinkles. There are many other reasons for these wrinkles to occur before time or be more pronounced. They are as listed below:

- ➢ Pollution
- ➢ Extensive exposure to the sun
- ➢ Lack of vitamin D3
- ➢ Excessive use of cosmetics
- ➢ Constant changing of creams and cosmetics
- ➢ Smoking

Areas Of The Skin Prone To Wrinkle Formation

The skin on the face is the most sensitive and thin when compared to the rest of the body. Hence, wrinkles on the face are quite common. Wrinkles around the eyes, on the forehead, and laugh lines or wrinkles around the mouth are very common. Neck wrinkles are as well seen where the skin tends to begin droopy with age. Wrinkles on the hand, chest, and feet also develop in due time.

Minimizing Wrinkles Through Lifestyle

1. Consume foods high in vitamin C. Incorporate different foods into your diet every day that contain high amounts of vitamin C. These will aid build collagen, which makes your skin look firmer. They can additionally shield your skin from ultraviolet light injury that causes wrinkling. Some examples of foods high in vitamin C include:

> Tomatoes
> Chili peppers
> Mango
> Strawberries
> Broccoli
> Pineapple

2. Boost your vitamin E intake with nuts. Consume a moderate quantity of nut as a snack rather than chips. These contain healthy fats and vitamin E, which can facilitate your skin retain wetness. It can also reduce the appearance of wrinkles and protect you from harmful UV rays. Select any of the following foods to get plenty of vitamin E:

> Walnuts
> Almonds
> Hazelnuts
> Peanuts
> Pistachios

3. Enjoy a massage. Stimulate your circulation and relax yourself with an expert massage or one you are doing yourself. This can enhance nutrients to the skin and reduce stress, both of which may not only whip off wrinkles, but can prevent them in the future.

- ➢ Locate a qualified massage therapist online or ask your doctor for a recommendation.
- ➢ Rub on a little quantity of your favorite lotion with firm but gentle pressure. Focus on the part particularly at risk of wrinkles, such as the neck, under the eyes, or your forehead.

4. Eat plenty of berries. Use a wide selection of colorful berries at most meals. These contain polyphenols and antioxidants that promote cell regeneration that will cut back the looks of wrinkles and forestall them within the future. Choose any of the following berries to reap their wrinkle-busting potential:

- ➢ Blueberries
- ➢ Raspberries
- ➢ Strawberries
- ➢ Blackberries
- ➢ Currants
- ➢ Pomegranate

5. Drink green or ginger tea. Both green tea and ginger tea are full of antioxidants that can slow the signs of aging. Drinking a cup of tea every day can be a great way to keep your skin looking beautiful while also getting some relaxation.

- ➢ You can mix honey into your ginger tea to add more anti-aging benefits, as well as a bit of sweetness.

> You can as well make a face mask utilizing green tea. Simply combine tea leaf powder into brewed white tea till it becomes a paste. Apply the paste to your skin, then rinse in 15 minutes.

6. Bananas

When we refer to a healthier diet, it is much more than just eating these nutritious foods. You can use these foods for topical application as well. Bananas can also be used for this purpose. Its nutritional properties fight the causes of wrinkles. Mash two bananas and form a paste. Now apply it on your face and allow it to sit for half an hour and then wash it off. You could also mix it with some avocado and honey for the same effect.

7. Egg whites

Eggs can do wonders for your overall health. For your skin, egg whites can serve as the natural remedy for your skin wrinkles. All you would like to try and do is make some egg whites in a bowl and apply it on your skin directly. Massage it lightly and permit it to sit for quarter-hour. You could also leave it on without any disturbance and wait for it to dry out. Then wash it with warm water. Protein, vitamin E, and B can cure those fine lines naturally.

8. Aloe vera

Aloe vera is rich in malic acid which improves skin elasticity. All you need to do is take some gel from the leave and apply it on your skin as it is. Wait for 15 minutes or till it dries and then wash it off. You could also mix the gel with some vitamin E oil and apply it on your face for the same effect.

9. Carrots

Carrots are rich in vitamin A which promotes collagen production, thereby keeping the skin smooth and wrinkle-free. For this, you can apply a carrot paste on your face every day. Just boil some carrots and blend it into a paste with some honey. Apply it on your face, rest for half an hour and then wash it off. You could also eat them raw.

Other Tips To Fight Wrinkles

1. Drink And Rinse

On an average, an adult is advised to drink at least 1 to 2 liters of water in a day. However, studies indicate that you should drink 5 to 6 liters of water in a day to keep your organs healthy. Drinking ample amount of water helps your body flush out toxic waste. A clean inside reflects on the body outside.

2. Trim Those Bangs

Trimming those bangs if you are over 25 is a sure way to help reduce the appearance of wrinkles on your forehead. A quick trim can gather your face, accentuate your features, and reduce wrinkles. Try it!

3. The Sun – The Ultimate Villain

Yes, the sun is the most crucial factor that contributes to the generation of wrinkles. The harmful UV rays of the sun are extremely damaging for the skin and can deplete it of its natural moisture. The weakened collagen fails to shield the skin from more injury. The risk of skin cancer also increases if you step out in the sun every day without any protection. So, do not forget to use an umbrella or a hat the next time you step out when the sun is intense.

4. Sleep

Nothing is more practical to ease out those fine lines showing on the skin. As you sleep, the body goes into the restoration mode, and at the same time, secretes the human growth hormone (HGH). HGH plays a quintessential role in keeping your skin more elastic and less prone to wrinkles. If your body is bereft of rest, it results in an increase in the production of cortisol, which breaks down the skin cells, triggering wrinkle formation. Make sure you sleep on your back. Sleeping on your sides can cause wrinkles on that side to increase.

5. De-stress

Lighten up, for stress will have adverse effects on your beauty. Stress, together with anxiety and tension, could make your skin thin and weaker and prone to wrinkles. Indulge in recreational activities so that stress does not get to you. Think about all the good things in your life – and smile. A smile can assist you beat the strain and banish those wrinkles.

Life often springs unexpected situations at you. You need to learn the technique of keeping calm, no matter how challenging or adverse the situation may be. Stay relaxed all the time, and maintain a healthy lifestyle.

6. Scarf Up

Non-radical problems, such as pollution, affect your skin the most. Use a scarf if you have to step out for long hours to protect your face from exposure to dust and pollution. Cleanse your skin with a gentle face wash replenished with antioxidants for dirt, grime, and wrinkle-free skin.

7. Soak In SPF

As mentioned previously, extensive exposure to the sun damages the skin beyond repairable levels. Studies suggest that while vitamin D is a blessing to the skin, exposing yourself to the ultraviolet-rich sun rays for a long time does more harm than good. It speed up skin aging, resulting in the early onset of wrinkles.

Be liberal while using sunscreen. Opt for a sunscreen that has high SPF. Also, choose a product that is water-based and does not contain harmful chemicals. Apply it even during cloudy days. Apply it at least 15 minutes before your tryst with the sun, and reapply every 4 to 6 hours.

8. Quit Smoking And Alcohol

Apart from being hazardous to your health, smoking can also cause wrinkles. The carcinogens in cigarettes act as a toxic plastic bag around your pretty face, blocking and depriving it of oxygen. This aggravates the appearance of wrinkles on your skin. So, say goodbye to smoking. It may sound stereotyped, yet, you should quit alcohol as soon as you can. If you are unable to resist alcohol completely, you should set a limit on the intake.

9. It Can Be The Genes Sometimes

Strange, but true. Wrinkles can be the result of several genetic factors. In some families, people look aged in their mid-40s. On the contrary, in another family, the members might look young even in their 70s. Therefore, you should consider the genetic factor as far as wrinkles are concerned. However, it does not necessarily imply that genetically driven wrinkles cannot be removed. You can still eliminate them with correct skin care procedures and solutions.

CHAPTER TWO

HOW TO OVERCOME BLEMISHES

What Are Blemishes?

Blemishes are imperfections that often appear on your face, including blackheads, whiteheads, uneven skin tone, dark spots, pigmentation, scars, and other marks and spots. Without the right treatment, they can often get worse, making you feel unattractive, as though you are lacking your natural glow.

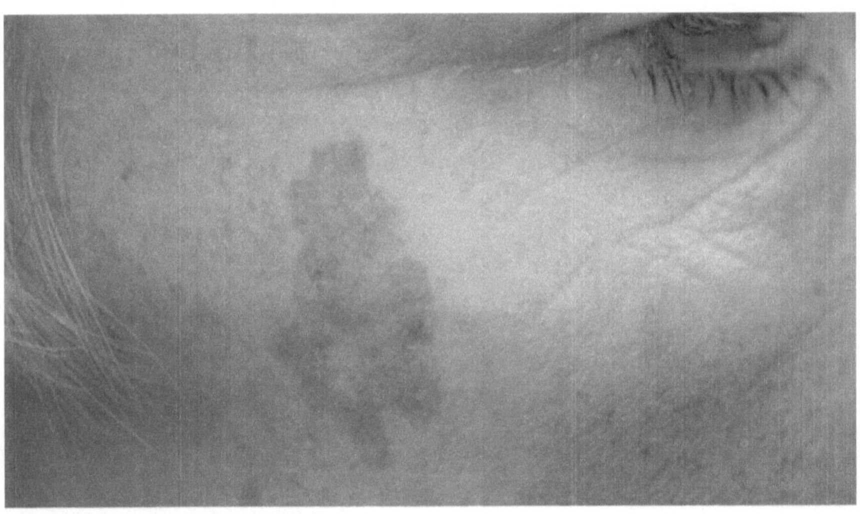

What Causes Blemishes?

Blemishes occur due to one major reason, and that is excessive oil production. They are primarily the consequence of an acne burst. The pimple goes away, but it leaves behind scars that will never let you forget it. The reason behind a blemish is the obstruction of pores with dead skin cells and excessive oil, which results in acne. When this happens in the upper layers of the epidermis, we get whiteheads and blackheads. However, when this happens in the inner layers, we end up with acne. Acne makes our skin red and inflamed, which then changes into a blemish once the pimple goes off. Obviously, waiting for the pimples to vanish and praying that blemishes do not appear is not the solution. Some things do not fix themselves, and pimples are one of them. Treating them appropriately is the only way you can make sure they do not come back to haunt you. Here is how you can remove blemishes (while treating acne) with wonderful secrets.

How to eliminate Blemishes

1. Baking Soda For Blemishes

You Will Need

> ➤ 1 teaspoon baking soda
> ➤ Water or olive oil

What You Have To Do

1. Add a few drops of water or olive oil to the baking soda and mix well to get a paste.

2. Apply this paste on the affected area and leave it on for 5-10 minutes.

3. Slowly scrub the paste off and rinse the area with clean water.

4. Repeat this twice a week.

Baking soda neutralizes the pH of the skin and also scrubs away the dead cells that have accumulated at the site of the blemish. This makes the blemish appear lighter, and after multiple usage, your blemish will completely vanish.

2. Egg White For Blemishes

You Will Need

> egg white
> A face pack brush (optional)

What You Have To Do

1. On clean skin, apply the egg white using either the brush or your fingers.

2. Let it dry for about 10 minutes.

3. Rinse it off with water.

4. Pat dry and apply a moisturizer.

5. Apply this face mask twice a week.

Egg white contains natural enzymes that tone the skin and lighten blemishes and scars .

3. Apple Cider Vinegar For Blemishes

You Will Need

- ➢ 1 part apple cider vinegar
- ➢ 8 parts water
- ➢ Spray bottle

What You Have To Do

1. Make a mix of the vinegar and water. Store the solution in the spray bottle.

2. Spritz your face with this and let it dry naturally.

3. Do this once or twice daily.

ACV works as an astringent and balances the skin's pH while killing the harmful microbes that may infect the pores. Its mild acids help to lighten blemishes. The excess oil production is also brought under control.

4. Make an Oatmeal Mask to Cleanse Your Skin

Oatmeal is proven to cleanse and soothe the skin while also helping blemished or damaged areas with its antioxidant properties. Create your mask by using rose water and 2 tablespoons of uncooked oats to create a paste. Add 1 drop or 2 of lemon juice to assist lighten your blemishes. Apply to your face liberally before leaving for about 10-12 minutes and rinsing off with warm water. This is suitable for using twice a week.

5. Use Shea Butter to Nourish Your Skin

Not only will shea butter work to nourish your skin but it will also help reduce the appearance of scars and blemishes with the vitamin A it contains. It also works to keep your skin looking smoother and younger. For a perfect result, use shea butter (the organic kind is best) each night, massaging it intensely into the target areas so your skin absorbs it completely. Leave it on when you go to bed so it can absorb further and work its magic.

6. Choose Tomato or Lemon Juice to Lighten Blemishes

Fresh lemon juice or tomato juice is great for helping lighten the appearance of blemishes. Lemon juice works like bleach (but far less harsh) on your skin, evening out your skin tone and reducing the appearance of scars and blemishes. Tomato juice as well can assist in taking away skin tan and blemishes with its antioxidant and antioxidants. Just take one tiny tomato to form a pulp and massage it into your face. You can use both of these every day; just apply to the necessary area for about 10 minutes before washing them off.

7. Use Honey to Improve the Health of Your Skin

Honey has an emollient and humectants property which means it is great at keeping your skin in tip-top condition, nourishing your skin cells. And with its antioxidants, it will additionally fade scars by substitution these cells with new, unmarred ones, removing free radicals from your skin. Just apply raw honey to your blemishes for 15 minutes each day, rinsing off with warm water. Honey can also be combined with lemon and other ingredients to create indulgent face masks.

HOW TO OVERCOME CELLULITE

What is cellulite?

Do you have uneven, lumpy skin on your hips, thighs, or buttocks? This may be a sign of cellulite. Cellulite happens when the skin covering certain areas of fat is pulled downward to the deeper tissues by the connective tissue bands. This creates an uneven surface.

Cellulite is commonly found on:

- ➢ hips
- ➢ thighs
- ➢ abdomen
- ➢ buttocks
- ➢ breasts

Cellulite affects ladies more than men because of the various fat, muscle, and connective tissue distribution. It is thought to affect 80% to 90% of women in varying degrees. Cellulite is not harmful.

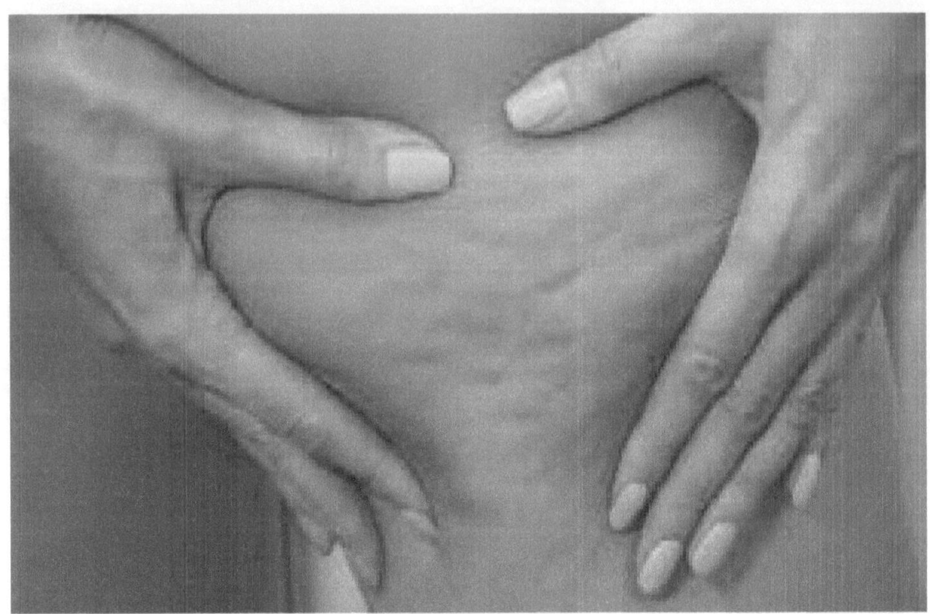

What causes cellulite?

Cellulite is caused by a buildup of fat beneath the skin. Some women are more predisposed to it than others. The amount of fatty tissue you have, and how obvious it is can be as a result of your genes, body fat percentage, and age. The thickness of your skin additionally affects the looks of cellulite. People of all body sorts and weights can have cellulite. The distribution of fat in ladies is a lot more visible than in men. The collagen fibers between the skin and muscle detach the underlying fat into multiple pockets. Cellulite will become a lot more visible as you age and your skin becomes slimmer and loses its elasticity. This exposes the rippled connective tissues underneath.

Cellulite may be caused by:

- ➢ hormones
- ➢ poor diet
- ➢ an unhealthy lifestyle
- ➢ accumulated toxins
- ➢ genetics
- ➢ weight gain
- ➢ inactivity
- ➢ pregnancy

Medical procedures for reducing cellulite

The following medical procedures can be performed by a doctor or dermatologist. Your healthcare provider can help you to determine which treatment is best for you.

Cryolipolysis

Cryolipolysis, or CoolSculpting, is a catching procedure that eliminates cellulite by freezing the fat cells underneath the skin. This causes the fat cells to rupture and their contents to be absorbed by the body. Several treatments are needed to dissolve an inch of fat. It may take three to four months to see a noticeable reduction in cellulite.

Ultrasound

Ultrasound could be a noninvasive procedure that uses sound waves to focus on and eliminate fat within the abdomen and thighs. Results take two or three months. It is recommended that you combine ultrasound with another cellulite treatment. You may also be able to use ultrasound to measure the effectiveness of other cellulite treatments.

Cellfina

Cellfina is a nonsurgical procedure. During the procedure, a needle is employed to break up the robust bands underneath the skin to get rid of fatty tissue (cellulite) on the thighs and buttocks. Results can be seen in as little as three days and can last up to three years.

Laser and radiofrequency treatments

These medical therapies use tissue massage with combinations of radio frequency technology, infrared light, and diode laser energy to treat cellulite. Heat and suctioning may also be used. Cellulaze is one sort of laser treatment that breaks up the robust bands underneath the skin that allows cellulite to be noticeable. It may also thicken your skin. Improvements are seen after a series of treatments, and can last six months or longer.

Vacuum-assisted precise tissue release

This procedure breaks up the robust bands underneath the skin with a tool containing tiny blades. The bands are been cut, which allows the tissue to move upward to fill in the dimpled skin.

Results may last up to three years.

Learn how to significantly reduce the appearance of cellulite with lifestyle changes, skincare products and special treatments.

Update Your Diet

1. Drink plenty of water. Hydrating your body keeps your skin cells look fresh and revived, which can reduce the appearance of cellulite. Drink at least 8 glasses of water a day to make sure your system is getting all the water it needs.

- ➢ Endeavor to drink a glass of water first thing in the morning, before intake of your morning coffee or tea.
- ➢ Convey one bottle of water with you as you go about your day. Always remember to refill it.

2. Eat fruits and vegetables. A diet stuffed with healthy fruits and vegetables can assist you to keep your weight down, and reduce the appearance of cellulite. Fruits and vegetables even have high water content, so they also help keep you hydrated.

- ➢ Have a spinach smoothie for breakfast. Blend 1 cup of almond milk, 1 cup of spinach, 1/2 a banana and a kiwi or handful of strawberries. This high-powered breakfast can keep your energy high, and it is a great way to get a serving of vegetables at breakfast.
- ➢ Eat plenty of raw vegetables. Raw salad greens, broccoli, carrots and other vegetables are packed with nutrients, antioxidants and water. If you create them to be the mainstay of your diet, you will see a distinction within the quantity of fatty tissue you have got.

3. Eat healthy fats. Cellulite is caused by the fat just below the skin, however if your skin is toned and healthy, the fatty tissue will not be as noticeable. Foods like olives, nuts, avocados, fish and oil comprises of omega-3 fatty acid, that are vital for healthy skin.

> ➢ Consume Omega-3 fatty acid. Since we have a tendency to eat fatty foods or a minimum of foods stuffed with all types of fats all the time, therefore, ingesting the correct fatty acids and neglecting those that are harmful to us are important for an entire recovery from cellulite. Pasture-raised meats, dairy products enriched with Omega-3, Edamame, wild rice, canola oil, or walnuts are only a few of the many foods that are rich in this fatty acid and should be consumed in much quantities for an entire removal of fatty tissue.

4. Avoid foods that lead to more cellulite. Foods that cause you to obtain weight and retain water increase the number of cellulite you have got. Avoid the subsequent foods to stop additional fatty tissue from appearing:

> ➢ Fried foods like onion rings French fries, and fried chicken.
> ➢ Packaged snacks like corn chips, potato chips, cheese puffs, and pretzels.
> ➢ Foods that are high in salt, like canned dips or soup and dressings, make you to retain water.
> ➢ Foods that are high in sugar, like baked goods, candy, and soda, make you to gain weight.

➢ Alcohol, especially when it is been paired with a sugary mixer like cranberry juice or soda, can enable you to gain weight and retain water.

Start a New Exercise Routine

1. Incorporate weight training. Weight coaching, in contrast to cardio exercises, tones the muscles under your skin and causes it to appear more firm. This can greatly reduce the appearance of cellulite.

➢ Buy free weights and perform exercises meant to tone your thighs, buttocks, and abs. If you have got fatty tissue on your arms, perform arm exercises as well.

➢ Join a gym and work with a trainer to increase the amount of weight you lift over time. Contrasting to common belief that lifting heavier weights fewer times, rather than doing so much of reps with lighter weights, is better for building muscle.

2. Do high intensity exercises. Pairing weight training with exercises that gets your heart pumping ends up creating lean muscle mass, which can cause your thighs and buttocks to appear smoother over time. Try the following exercises after doing a light warm-up:

➢ Do outdoor sprints. Measure out a distance of 1/4 mile (0.4 km) on your street or at a nearby park. Sprint that distance, take a break for about 20 seconds, sprint it again, and repeat for a total of about 4 sprints. As you improve, add additional sprints to your physical training.

> Sprint on your treadmill. If you work out indoors, use a faster setting on your treadmill to sprint for about 3 minutes. Increase the speed as you improve over time.

> Do bike sprints. Using either your bicycle or a stationary bike, ride as quick as you will uphill for a couple of minutes.

Try a New Skincare Regimen

1. Start dry brushing your skin. Dry brushing improves your circulation and helps your skin eliminate toxins, reducing the appearance of cellulite. Buy a body brush created with natural fibers and include dry brushing to your morning routine.

> Ensure your skin and the brush are both dry before beginning.

> Beginning at your feet, brush upward toward your heart. Concentrate on areas with a lot of cellulite, like your thighs and buttocks. Brush your arms from your hands to your shoulders. Brush your abdomen in a clockwise manner and your arms in an upward motion. All brushing movements ought to be created towards your heart to encourage the comeback of blood and lymphatic flow.

> Have a shower after brushing to wash out the dead skin cells and toxins that have risen to the surface.

2. Improve your skin tone. Taking measures to make your skin look tight and healthy does not actually get rid of cellulite, but it can go a long way toward temporarily reducing its appearance. Try the following techniques:

- Bathe in cool water or lukewarm, rather than hot water. Cool water tightens your skin and makes it look more toned.

- Moisturize your skin with a product that contains caffeine. Buy a cream or lotion that contains a minimum of 5% caffein, which is said to improve skin tone and decrease the appearance of cellulite.

- Utilize another topical product designed to minimize the appearance of cellulite. There exist several creams and lotions in the market that are designed specifically for this purpose.

CHAPTER THREE

HOW TO OVERCOME ECZEMA

Eczema is said to be a condition where patches of skin become inflamed, red, itchy, cracked, and rough. Blisters may sometimes occur. Different stages and kinds of skin disorder (Eczema) have an effect on 31.6% of persons in the United States. The word "eczema" is as well used specifically to speak regarding atopic dermatitis, the most common type of eczema. "Atopic" refers to a collection of diseases involving the system, including asthma, hay fever, and atopic dermatitis. Dermatitis is an inflammation of the skin. Some individuals outgrow the condition, whereas others can still have it throughout adulthood.

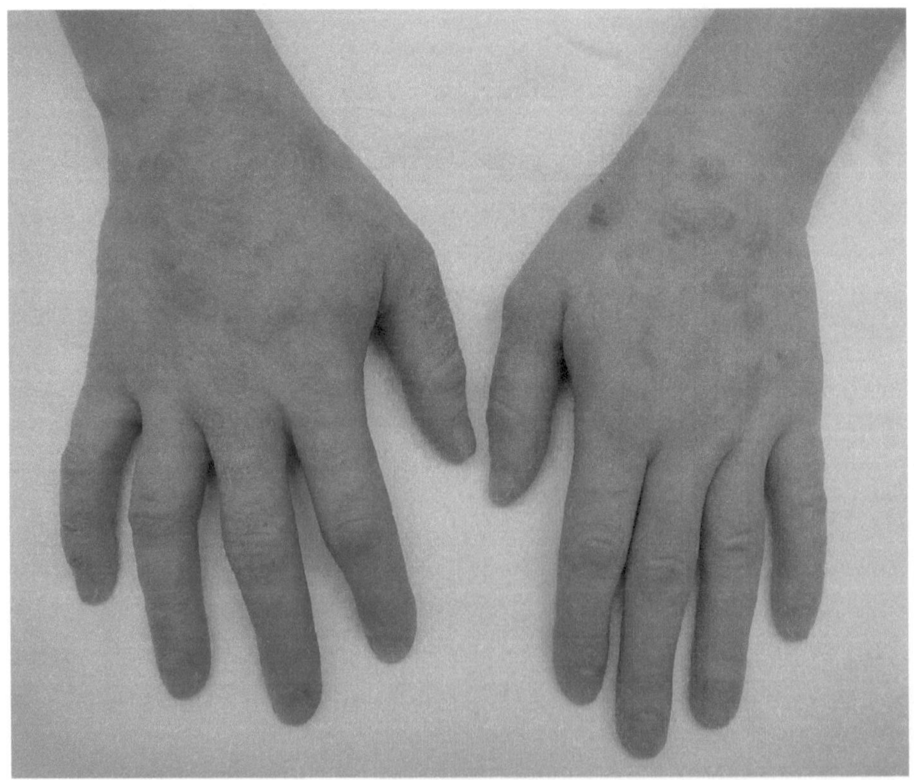

Symptoms in adults

> ➢ Rashes commonly appear in wrinkles of the knees or elbows or the nape of the neck.
> ➢ Rashes cover much of the body.
> ➢ Rashes can be especially prominent on the neck, face, and around the eyes.
> ➢ Rashes can cause very dry skin.
> ➢ Rashes can be permanently itchy.
> ➢ Rashes in adults can be more scaly than those occurring in children.
> ➢ Rashes can lead to skin infections.

Adults who developed atopic dermatitis as a child but no longer experience the condition may still have dry or easily-irritated skin, hand eczema, and eye problems. The appearance of skin suffering from dermatitis can depend upon what proportion an individual scratches and whether or not the skin is infected. Scratching and rubbing also irritate the skin, increase inflammation, and make itchiness worse.

Types

There are many different types of eczema. While this book has focused mainly on atopic dermatitis, other types include:

> ➢ **Allergic contact dermatitis:** This is a skin reaction following contact with a substance or allergen that the immune system recognizes as foreign.

- ➤ **Dyshidrotic eczema:** This is an irritation of the skin on the palms of the hands and the soles of the feet. It is characterized by blisters.

- ➤ **Neurodermatitis:** This forms scaly patches of skin on the head, forearms, wrists, and lower legs. It is caused by a localized itch, such as an insect bite.

- ➤ **Nummular eczema:** it appears as circular patches of irritated skin that can be crusted, itchy, and scaly.

- ➤ **Stasis dermatitis:** This is a skin irritation of the lower leg usually related to circulatory problems.

Causes

The specific cause of eczema remains unknown, but it is believed to develop due to a combination of genetic and environmental factors. Eczema is not contagious. Children are more likely to develop eczema if a parent has had the condition or another atopic disease. If both parents have an atopic disease, the risk is even greater.

Environmental factors are also known to bring out the symptoms of eczema, such as:

- ➤ **Irritants:** These include soaps, detergents, shampoos, disinfectants, juices from fresh fruits, meats, or vegetables.

- ➤ **Allergens:** mold, pollens, pets, Dust mites, and dandruff can result to eczema.

- ➢ **Microbes:** These include bacteria such as Staphylococcus aureus, viruses, and certain fungi.
- ➢ **Hot and cold temperatures:** Very hot or cold weather, high and low humidity, and perspiration from exercise can bring out eczema.
- ➢ **Foods:** Dairy products, eggs, nuts and seeds, soy products, and wheat can cause eczema flare-ups.
- ➢ **Stress:** This is an indirect cause of eczema and can make the symptoms worse.
- ➢ **Hormones:** Women can go through increased eczema symptoms at times when their hormone levels are varying, for instance during pregnancy and at certain points in the menstrual cycle.

Eczema will have an effect on folks of all ages and might cause quite little bit of misery. Doctors often prescribe a steroidal cream. For many people, steroids may have unwanted side effects, and this treatment does not always work very well. The good news is that there are different stuff you will do to ease the skin sensation, dryness, and skin changes. Implementing some natural remedies could create a big distinction in how your skin appears and feels. If your skin does not respond to natural treatments or gets worsened, consider seeing your doctor.

NATURAL REMEDIES

There are various things that individuals with skin disease will do to support skin health and alleviate symptoms, such as:

- ➢ taking lukewarm baths

- ➢ Apply moisturizer within 3 minutes after bathing to "lock in" moisture
- ➢ moisturizing every day
- ➢ wearing cotton and soft fabrics, and avoiding rough, scratchy fibers and tight-fitting clothing
- ➢ utilizing a mild soap or a non-soap cleanser when washing
- ➢ try and avoid rapid changes of temperature and activities that enables you to sweat
- ➢ learning and avoiding individual eczema triggers
- ➢ utilizing a humidifier in dry or cold weather
- ➢ keeping fingernails short to prevent scratching from breaking the skin

HOW TO OVERCOME ACNE

What Causes Acne?

Acne begins when the pores in your skin get clogged with oil and dead skin cells. Each pore is connected to an oil gland (sebaceous gland), which produces an oily substance called sebum. Additional sebum will plug up pores, causing the growth of bacteria known as Propionibacterium acnes, or P. acnes. Your white blood cells attack P. acnes, leading to skin inflammation and acne. Some cases of acne are more severe than others, but common symptoms include whiteheads, blackheads and pimples. Many factors contribute to the event of acne, including stress, diet, genetics, hormone changes and infections.

Pimples, also called acne, are caused by a complex interplay of several factors, such as bacteria, hormonal changes, or clogged follicles on your skin. Certain types of bacteria can grow in these follicles, causing inflammation. While you will attempt to forestall or eliminate pimples, people often need to cope with them at some point. If you have acne, the healthiest thing you can do is to bring up your self-confidence. The Conventional acne treatment is costly and most times have undesirable side effects such as redness and irritation. This has prompted many of us to look for ways to treat acne naturally at home. The internet is crammed with suggestions , however do natural treatments truly work?

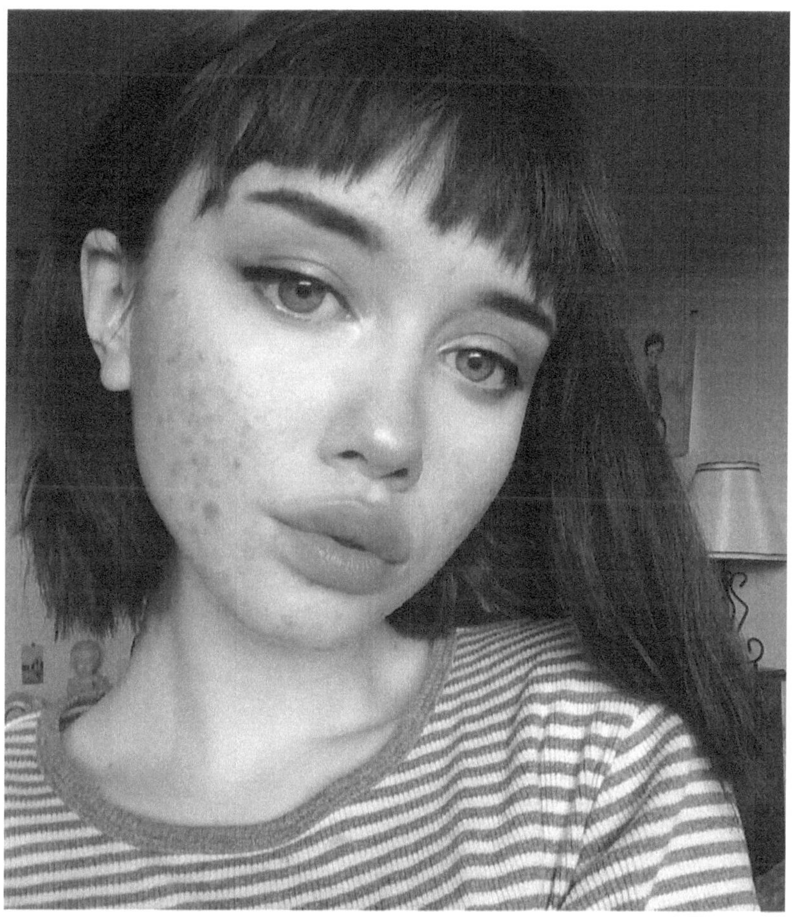

you might want to try.

Below are some home remedies for acne that

1. Take a Zinc Supplement

Zinc is a vital nutrient that is important for cell growth, hormone production, metabolism and immune function. It is additionally one of the most studied natural treatments for skin condition (acne). Research indicates that individuals with acne tend to possess lower levels of Zinc in their blood more than those with clear skin. Several studies have indicated that taking Zinc orally helps cut back acne. In one study, 48 persons suffering from acne were given oral Zinc supplements 3 times per day. After about 8 weeks, 38 patients experience 80–100% reduction in acne. The best dose of Zinc for acne has not been established, however many studies have shown a big reduction of acne utilizing 30–45 mg of elemental Zinc each day. Elemental Zinc refers to the quantity of Zinc that is present in the compound.

2. Make a Honey and Cinnamon Mask

These are 2 medications normally used for acne that are common for the skin that have antibacterial properties. Both honey and cinnamon are wonderful sources of antioxidants. Studies have found out that applying antioxidants to the skin is more practical at reducing acne than retinoids and benzyl peroxide. The antioxidants studied were nutrition B3, linoleic (omega-6) fatty acid and sodium ascorbyl phosphate (SAP), which happens to be a vitamin C derivative. These specific antioxidants are not found in honey or cinnamon; however there is a possibility that alternative antioxidants might have an analogous impact. Honey and cinnamon also possess the ability to fight microorganism and cut back inflammation, which are 2 factors that trigger acne. While the antioxidant, anti-inflammatory, and antibacterial properties of honey and cinnamon might profit acne-prone skin, no studies exist on their ability to treat acne.

How to Make a Honey and Cinnamon Mask

1. Mix 2 tablespoons honey and 1 teaspoon cinnamon together to form a paste.

2. After the cleansing, apply the mask to your face and leave it on for about 10–15 minutes.

3. The mask should be rinsed off completely and pat your face dry.

3. Spot Treat With Tea Tree Oil

Tea tree oil is a vital oil that is extracted from the leaves of Melaleuca alternifolia, a little tree native to Australia. It is renowned for its ability to fight microorganism and cut back skin inflammation. What's additional, several studies indicate that applying 5% tea tree oil to the skin effectively reduces acne. When compared to 5 percent benzoyl peroxide, 5 percent tea tree oil failed to act as quickly, however it did considerably improve acne after a period of about 3 months of use. It as well resulted in fewer adverse effects like irritation, dryness and burning, compared to benzoyl peroxide. Tea tree oil is incredibly potent, so always dilute it before applying it to your skin.

How to Use It

1. Mix a part tea tree oil with 9 parts water

2. Dip a cotton swab into the mixture and apply it to affected areas.

3. Apply moisturizer if desired.

4. Repeat this process 1–2 times per day, as needed.

4. Moisturize With Aloe Vera

Aloe vera is said to be a tropical plant whose leaves manufactures a transparent gel. The gel is often added to lotions, creams, ointments and soaps. It is commonly used to treat abrasions, rashes, burns and other skin conditions. When it is applied to the skin, aloe vera gel can assist in healing wounds, treat burns and fight inflammation. Aloe vera also comprises of salicyclic acid and sulfur, which are both used extensively in the treatment of acne. Several studies have indicated that applying salicyclic acid to the skin considerably reduces acne. In like manner, applying sulfur has been established to be a great acne treatment. While research shows great promise, the anti-acne benefits of aloe vera itself require further scientific evidence.

How to Use It

1. The gel should be scraped from the aloe plant out with a spoon.

2. The gel should be applied directly to clean skin as a moisturizer.

3. Repeat 1–2 times per day, or as desired.

You can conjointly purchase Aloe vera gel from the shop, but make sure it is pure aloe without any added ingredients.

5. Take a Fish Oil Supplement

Omega-3 fatty acids are incredibly healthy fats that offer a multitude of health benefits. You must obtain these fats from your diet, but research indicates that most persons who eat a standard Western diet do not get enough of them. Fish oils comprises of 2 main forms of omega-3 fatty acids: eicosapentaenoic acid (EPA) and docosahexaenoic (DHA). EPA profits the skin in many ways, as well as managing production, maintaining adequate hydration and preventing skin condition (acne).

6. Exfoliate Regularly

Exfoliation is a way of removing the top layer of dead skin cells. It may be mechanically achieved by utilizing a brush or scrub to physically take away the cells. Alternatively, it may be removed with chemicals by applying an acid that can dissolve them. Exfoliation is believed to boost acne by removing the skin cells that clog up pores. It is additionally believed to make acne treatments for the skin more effective by permitting them to penetrate deeper, once the top layer of skin is been removed. Unfortunately, the analysis on exfoliation and its ability to treat skin disorder is restricted. Some studies show that microdermabrasion, that could be a methodology of exfoliation, will improve the skin's look, together with some cases of skin disorder scarring.

How to Make a Scrub at Home

1. Mix equal parts sugar (or salt) and coconut oil.

2. Scrub skin with mixture and rinse well.

3. Exfoliate as regularly as desired up to once each day.

7. Apply Green Tea to Your Skin

Green tea is incredibly high in antioxidants, and drinking it will promote healthiness. There are no studies exploring the advantages of drinking green tea once it involves acne, however applying it on to the skin has been shown to assist. This is likely due to the fact that, the flavonoids and tannins in green tea are known to assist in the fight against bacteria and scale back inflammation, which are two main causes of acne. The major antioxidant in green tea — epigallocatechin-3-gallate (EGCG) — has been shown to reduce sebum production, fight inflammation and inhibit the growth of P. acnes in individuals with acne-prone skin. Multiple studies have shown that applying a 2–3% tea extract to the skin considerably reduces sebum production and pimples in those with acne. You can obtain creams and lotions that contain tea, however it is even as straightforward to form your own mixture at home.

How to Use It

1. Immerse green tea in boiling water for 3–4 minutes.

2. Allow tea to cool.

3. employing a cotton ball, apply tea to skin or pour into a spray bottle to spray it on the skin.

4. Allow it to dry, and then use water to rinse and pat dry.

You can additionally add the remaining tea leaves to honey and create a mask. Even though there is not any proof that drinking green tea will fight acne, some research suggests it may still be beneficial. For example, drinking tea has been shown to lower blood glucose and insulin levels that are factors which will contribute to the development of acne.

8. Reduce Stress

The hormones discharged during times of stress might increase secretion production (sebum) and skin inflammation, making skin disorder (acne) worse. In fact, multiple studies have connected stress to a rise in acne severity. What is additional, stress can slow wound healing by up to 40%, which may slow the repair of acne lesions. Certain relaxation and stress-reduction treatments are indicated to boost acne, but more research needs to be done.

Ways to Reduce Stress

➢ Get more sleep

> Engage in physical activity

> Practice yoga

> Meditate

> Take deep breaths

CHAPTER FOUR

BEAUTY ANTI AGING SECRET

Our dream is to age like a fine wine. So, I did some questioning by asking specialists such as dermatologists, nutritionists, and makeup artists for their secrets to younger-looking skin, voluminous hair, eating well, and more so you can look and feel your best for years to come. The following are natural anti-aging secret:

1. Olive Oil

The anti-aging properties of olive oil can be trailed to the polyphenols and monounsaturated fatty acid (oleic acid) in it. Powered with monounsaturated fats and Vitamins B and D, it not only stops the appearance of new wrinkles, but also eliminates existing ones.

How to use: Mix 1 spoon of olive oil with one spoon of lemon juice and then apply it to your face. Leave for about 10 minutes and wash off. This will assist you in preventing the appearance of wrinkles.

2. Lemon Juice

Lemon juice contains alpha acid, a common ingredient in anti-ageing treatments which helps peel away the layer of dead skin cells.

How to use: combine juice with sugar crystals to make an exfoliating scrub for your hands. Remember, your hands age faster than your face.

3. Avocado

This super fruit when applied to dry skin, assist in lubricating the skin. Their high levels of fats and vitamins such as A, D and E help the skin to retain moisture and work as anti-agers.

How to use: include the fruit as often times as possible as a part of your diet.

4. Aloe

Together with carotene and Vitamins C and E, which aid in keeping skin plum, this ingredient is a regular in most anti-aging potions.

How to use: Cut and peel an aloe vera leaf to show the gel win it, and then apply to skin. Also, drink a little glass of natural aloe vera juice 2 times weekly.

5. Cucumber

High in water content and packed with nutrients such as vitamins A and E magnesium, potassium, cucumbers fosters blood circulation and healing, which assist in the reduction of wrinkles around the eyes and makes for a glowing complexion.

How to use: Place cucumber slices over your eyes to depuff. You can additionally juice a cucumber and add a couple of drops of honey to create a soothing, hydrating face mask.

6. Green Tea

That green tea is a good weight loss solution is very popular. However, what you might not have known is that green tea is rich in antioxidants known as EGCG, which assist in battling with wrinkles and increases cell turnover.

How to use: Brew a cup of tea leaf on mild heat; wait for it to heat up. Soak a face cloth and place it over your eyes. The heat can open up pores and therefore the tea can infuse itself into your skin. Its anti-aging properties can help deflate bags underneath the eyes while treating the rest of your face.

7. Ginger

A common ingredient found in the kitchen, ginger is rich in an antioxidant known as gingerol, which has been proven to protect against collagen breakdown.

How to use: begin the day with a cup of hot tea with cut ginger and a small unspecified quantity of honey for optimum anti-ageing benefits to the skin.

8. Banana

There is a lot more a banana will do than just fill you up at breakfast. It is as well known to spice up collagen production and known to keep skin aging at bay.

How to use: to create a banana anti-wrinkle mask, take a ripe banana and blend it with honey. Apply on your face. Allow it to dry. Wash off with heat water, and notice the tightness in your skin in 4-weeks flat.

9. Orange

Together with vitamin c, which is a naturally brightener, citrus fruits can be a great way to keep ageing at bay. They assist in cleansing you from the inner body out by removing toxins and impurities that would appear on your face.

How to use: Utilize a slice of orange in a face pack made with created oatmeal and honey for larger benefits. Or simply soak a bit of cotton in a bowl of handmade orange juice, wipe your face with it, and notice the brightness over a period.

OTHER TIPS INCLUDE:

Use Primer First

Skin thins and dries with age, so lines and wrinkles start to appear. Applying primer before you place on your makeup helps minimize the looks of fine lines and pores by filling them in. This way your skin may be a sleek blank canvas for you to use your makeup. Skin primer does not remove fine lines and huge pores, but it can aid both to appear less visible. Silicone is said to be a common ingredient in skin primer that works well for the aim.

Make Sure You Can See

Eyesight tends to decline with age. Most persons need glasses when they get up to 40 years. Your inability to see well could have an effect on your ability to be precise once applying makeup. No one wants to look like a clown! Invest in a unique magnifying mirror and use it while applying your makeup, especially eyeliner, eye shadow, and mascara. A magnifying mirror is as well a really important tool to have on hand when you are grooming or filling in eyebrows. See your ophthalmologist for regular eye exams to make sure you have an adequate prescription for your eyeglasses or contact lenses so you can see clearly.

Make Your Eyes Pop

Eyelids get droopy as we age, and eyelashes and eyebrows may become more sparse. Draw attention to your best features. Apply eyeliner in a color that makes your eyes pop. Apply a skinny line of eyeliner along your upper and lower lash lines. This will enable your eye lashes appear thicker. Use a complementary color of eye shadow on your upper lid. Use softer reminder eye shadow as you grow old, and apply least product.

Skip Thick Foundation

Foundation is nice for making your skin tone seem even and sleek. It will hide imperfections such as scars, freckles, age spots, and other skin problem issues but, if you apply foundation too thick or too heavy, it can actually make you appear older due to the fact that it sinks into lines and wrinkles, making them seem worse. Here is the right way to apply foundation. First, clean and dry your face. Next, apply moisturizer appropriate for your skin type. Then, apply primer. Now you are ready to apply foundation. Use a light touch together with a sponge applicator to dab the product over your entire face. The color should be blended fastidiously on the sides of your face and at the jaw line. By so doing, you prevent possessing a severe line between skin areas in the absence of foundation. Apply foundation sparingly. A little goes a long way.

Fill in Sparse Eyebrows

Eyebrows tend to become thinner and grey as we come of age. Since eyebrows frame the face, their appearance determines how youthful you look. Fill in and darken aging eyebrows. Utilize an eyebrow pencil which approximates your hair color to fill in distributed areas. Make use of eyebrow powder over pencil in areas to make the color set. Avoid utilizing colors which are a lot darker than your hair color. Eyebrows that are very dark can look unnatural and can make you look aged.

ADVANTAGES AND DISADVANTAGES ASSOCIATED WITH ORGANIC AND INORGANIC SKIN CARE MANAGEMENT

Would you accept that oils in their purest form can heal every skin woe; dehydration, irritation, sensitivity, aging, even oily. What we feed our skin matters. We all come from and are made of natural matter, so it should be no surprise that skincare should also be derived from the earth. Organic skincare are products that use organic ingredients that have gone through the growth process without the use of herbicides, pesticides or any other preservative. Natural products are very beneficial to the skin in more ways than one and though they may not be as mainstream as brands that hold more synthetic ingredients, organic skincare packs an enormous punch once it involves keeping your skin healthy.

Organic skin care holds a bunch of advantages, which has the usage of natural product that work for, rather than working against the skin. By using skincare products that are free from preservatives and artificial ingredients, you are as well helping your skin to repair itself.

Advantages Of Organic Skincare

1. Organic products are non-allergenic

Without harsh chemicals, organic skin care products are less likely to cause allergic reactions, inflammations or irritations. If an allergic reaction arises with the use of organic products, it would most likely be because of the natural ingredient (such as peanuts or strawberries), which would be easier to fish out.

2. Going organic is better for your skin

The artificial ingredients found in non-organic products could also be quick acting, but they are also invasive, causing harm that cannot be seen. Their chemical ingredients may provide instant gratification and visible results, but most of these only help you aesthetically by smoothening out wrinkles, removing sunspots, and diminishing blemishes. With prolonged usage, these chemicals may harm and weaken your skin as your body tries to cope with these foreign substances. As a result, oxygen exchange to the skin is reduced, causing premature aging and increased risk of developing sunspots.

3. Organic skin care products are made of natural ingredients

Reading through the ingredients label of any organic skin care product, you would most likely acknowledge most, if not all, of the items present. Certified organic merchandise are derived from plants and various natural occurring ingredients. More importantly, those organic ingredients are grown with no use of herbicides, synthetic fertilizers, pesticides, genetically modified organisms (GMOs), and other additives or chemicals. With that, you will make certain your skin and body absorb solely real, natural ingredients that are not harmful.

4. Organic skin care products work better

Plants grown organically are discovered to contain a top level of important antioxidant vitamins than non-organic plants. Because they are grown without herbicides and pesticides, their organic ingredients are also free from that contamination, which means the same for your skin and body. Also, up to 95 percent of organic skin care product's contents contain active ingredients while in artificial skin care products, active ingredients only make up 5 to 10% of its contents.

5. You are helping to preserve the environment

Because organic products use naturally grown ingredients that are free from toxic pesticides and fertilizers, they do not leave a harmful footprint on the planet, particularly the soil, water, and air. Organic farming is also better for wildlife, causes lower pollution from pesticide and fertilizer sprays, and produces less carbon dioxide and less dangerous wastes. By utilizing organic skin care product, you are helping to minimize your environmental impact and support the sustainability of our environment.

6. You are supporting cruelty-free skin care products

The beauty industry has received backlash for conducting animal testing for their products to ensure that they are safe for human use. Organic merchandise do not need to, because, with natural ingredients, they are safe and harm free! When you purchase organic skin care merchandise, you are buying cruelty-free skin care products and as well supporting the move towards abolishing animal testing in the industry.

Disadvantages

Sometimes even though the product is natural, this does not mean that it is purely organic. Natural merchandise are those merchandise that do not have any chemical or artificial ingredients in it. Organic products are products that have gone through a process to ensure that it is pure.

However organic products are only 95% pure. Some natural fragranced products have a chemical called phthalate which will lead to health and allergy issues. You will need to stay away from any product that mentions parfum or fragrance in order to maintain a safe side. Some natural products might have unsafe reactions to your body which will cause complications to your health. Ensure that what you use for your body and face is filled with natural ingredients that will not cause you any harm.

ADVANTAGES OF INORGANIC SKINCARE

> - Skin condition is often improved by the application of preventative and treatment cosmetics. This includes moisturizers, tone, wrinkle and blemish reduction cosmetics related to skin aging.
> - Symptoms of acne can be reduced.
> - Skins are often protected against sun burns by the right usage of sunscreen products.
> - Antiperspirants and Deodorants are effective in reducing perspiration and body odours.
> - Skin Fragrance is often used to elicit sturdy positive feeling.
> - Shaded merchandise – color cosmetics like lipstick, foundation, eye, nail and lip products are used to enhance the appearance.

DISADVANTAGES

Government regulations allow any type of ingredient to be used by the manufacturing companies of skin care, hair care and nail care products.

This is risky for the people utilizing these unknown and could be toxic ingredients. It is for this reason that people are encouraged to search the computer or go to the local library and look for options which are healthier. In the USA, it is the Food and Drug Administration (FDA) which regulates the rules and standards regarding the manufacture of food and drugs. However, the matter with this agency is that they do not particularly pay abundant attention to the makers of makeup and different skin care merchandise.

This practice allows the use of harmful chemicals in creating almost every kind of skin care product in the market. Some of the harmful ingredients that are explicitly used by skin product manufacturing companies are as follows: dioxane, DEA, mercury, nitrosamines, ammonium laureth sulfate, cyclomethicone, polyethylene glycol and polyethylene eth. These compounds when applied to the skin are usually easily absorbed and it has to be noted that a person's body has no way of getting the harmful ingredients out of its system. These toxins tend to reside in your intestine and will eventually spread throughout the entire body. This could then result to the damage of the various organs in your body.

CHAPTER FIVE

HOW TO BE NATURALLY BEAUTIFUL WITHOUT MAKEUP

Naturalness has consistently been in trend. Do you pay hours on a daily basis before the mirror to appear beautiful? While makeup is a fun way of expressing yourself and enhancing your features, you do not need to rely on it as a crush to define your beauty. A bare, natural look not solely permits your genuineness to shine through but it is additionally the simplest thing you will be able to carry around. Sincerely speaking, it is all about your insides and how well you look after yourself. Yes! You need to be mindful of essential aspects of your diet, your habits, your lifestyle and your skincare routine. If you have got even one among these parts ruined, the effects will inevitably reflect on your health and your overall appearance. Below are simple tips to looking beautiful without applying any lipstick, eye shadows, foundation, etc.

1. Sleep In Peace

A good night sleep goes hand-in-hand with the way you look and feel. It is crucial because your body repairs itself when you are asleep. Just like you would like to charge your telephone, your body needs to charge itself and to go through the day with your battery at 50 percent, only leads to added strain and inefficiency. 6-8 hours of quality sleep is significant for you to awaken feeling and looking nice. By doing this, you may have a glowing complexion, less of those dreaded dark circles under your eyes and you will slow down your aging process. The skin produces new collagen when you sleep. Do not let something in the world come in between you and your beauty sleep.

2. Make your eyebrows look perfect

On a face without any makeup, the eyebrows inevitably appear to be the center of attention. Shapen your eyebrows for your face shape. If desired, the eyebrows should be tinted with henna or dye. When selecting the color, make sure it matches your hair color. If you were not given birth to with thick brows, apply a mixture of castor oil and vitamin A to your eyebrows each day. After some weeks, you will notice the amazing transformation of your eyebrows.

3. Be Ingredient Conscious

Ingredient-conscious beauty is a thing; Yes! Just like what you put inside your body affects your overall health, what you put on the surface does the same. Your skin absorbs 60 percent of the stuff you put on so make sure you do some research on the ingredients that are present in your skin care, hair care, and beauty products. Stay clear from products that contain parabens, petrochemicals, and sulfates that may cause irritation to your skin or make your hair dry and frizzy. It is best to stick to products that contain natural ingredients.

4. Accentuate your eyes

To make your appearance "wider," your eyelashes should be curled with an eyelash curler, and then apply transparent gel to them. You can even go further and get eyelash extensions. Get rid of dark circles under your eyes. Start by reconsidering your diet. Dark circles may be the results of a deficiency of iron or B vitamins in your body (liver and red meat contains huge quantity of these). Choose eye creams with a whitening effect or the ones with retinol. Cold compresses with mint or green tea are very useful too.

5. Exfoliation Is Key

Make exfoliation a vital part of your skincare regime. It indeed is the key to radiant skin. Your skin is always shedding dead cells from the surface which helps in renewing itself with fresh and healthy cells. Give this natural process a helping hand by using a mild exfoliator. An excess of dead cells sitting on the surface of your skin can result to clogged pores, blackheads, acne and pimples. When you inculcate exfoliation into your regime, your serums and moisturizers are better absorbed into the skin making them work more efficiently. Opt for gentle scrubs or create your own natural scrubs at home using ingredients like gram flour or a coffee scrub. Keep exfoliation to at least 2 times in a week. You will see visible improvement within the health of your skin; it will appear more fresh and smooth.

6. Whiten your teeth

A bright smile adds a hundred points to any image. Therefore, ensure that nothing prevents you from appearing attractive. Utilize whitening toothpaste, especially after drinking coffee or wine. But remember not to overuse it as such toothpaste can be quite harsh. If your teeth are naturally grey or yellow, get them professionally whitened.

7. Take good care of your hair

Dull hair color and a haircut that was done some time ago are very not helpful for your makeup-free face. Choose simple hair styles and natural colors, as more drastic options would be discordant with a natural appearance. Get your split ends cut often, use products with heat protection, and do not go overboard with the styling products. Coconut oil can add shine to your hair. It also helps to fight dandruff, dryness, and other problems. Rinsing your hair with heated herbal extracts (sage and oak bark for brunettes, herbaceous plant and linden for blondes) as well makes your hair appear shinier.

8. Make Sunscreen Mandatory

Sunscreen is not an option. The Sun's UVA, UVB and UVC rays are the primary cause of premature aging of the skin. If you follow this easy step, you will thank yourself in the future. It helps prevent dark spots and hyper-pigmentation. SPF which is the 'sun protection factor' determines how well the sunscreen will protect you. Dermatologists suggest that you just wear a minimum of an SPF 30 before stepping out.

9. Find your own color

Correctly selecting the colour of your garments can assist in making your skin tone look even, hide flaws, and make your appearance more expressive. Skin with no foundation appears paler, and that is the reason it is necessary not to make things worse by selecting too dark and cold shades. White is also not the best option. The best ones are pure bright colors: blue, turquoise, emerald, peach. Ideally, you need to work out your color sort and make your choice according to specific rules.

Bust The Stress

In the recent lifestyle, we tend to all have crazy schedules and stress comes naturally. However, uncontrolled stress can lead to problems like headaches and hypertension. It can also lead to acne, hair fall and graying of hair. These are only a few severe outcomes of stress. So while you cannot entirely avoid bills, work, your life and all the stress that comes with it, you should find a way to manage it. Meditate, drink a nice hot cup of tea, listen to music or make some time for anything you love. Do take a chill pill now and then.

CONCLUSION

We value ourselves and create images of ourselves based largely on how other people see us. Whether it is counting the likes on our selfies or how many compliments we get on a night out, we rely on other people for their approval; but the natural way to go is to just accept yourself. Make a pact with yourself to believe in your beauty and accept it as it comes no matter what other people might think or say. That is when you can really start feeling beautiful. Also, a big part of being beautiful is taking good care of your body. That means truly taking care of it. Eating delicious, nutritious food that gives your body energy. Drinking enough water to keep you hydrated. Staying active so that your metabolism works normally and you keep your muscles strong.

Putting body milk all over yourself after a shower to show your skin some love. Putting on face and hair masks to really make a difference. It is those things that will not only make you look more beautiful, but feel more beautiful. As long as you are taking good care of yourself and doing your best; whatever your best might be that day, you will never have a reason not to feel beautiful. And do not forget that your mental health deserves just as much attention as your physical health. I strongly believe that this guide book "NATURAL BEAUTY FOR WOMEN" has gone a long way in explaining all you need to know. Practice what you have read and watch your life transform for good.

REFERENCES

- https://www.stylecraze.com/articles/effective-home-remedies-for-wrinkle-free-skin/#gref
- https://www.tatcha.com/blog/How-to-determine-your-skin-type.html
- https://www.wikihow.com/Get-Rid-of-Wrinkles-Naturally#relatedwikihows
- https://timesofindia.indiatimes.com/life-style/beauty/5-best-ways-to-remove-blemishes-naturally/photostory/63798245.cms?picid=63798520
- https://www.webmd.com/beauty/whats-your-skin-type#2
- https://bewellcompany.com/blogs/healthy-skincare/7-reasons-why-organic-skin-care-products-are-better-for-you
- https://www.stylecraze.com/articles/get-rid-of-blemishes/#gref
- https://www.onhealth.com/content/1/anti_aging_secrets
- https://brightside.me/inspiration-girls-stuff/10-simple-rules-for-looking-great-without-makeup-292560/
- http://biomoisturizing.com/beauty-products/76/
- https://www.healthyway.com/content/natural-beauty-meaning/
- https://janssencosmeticswest.com/blogs/default-blog/going-organic-the-advantages-of-natural-vs-inorganic-skincare
- https://www.wikihow.life/Deal-With-Pimples
- https://www.healthline.com/health/cellulite
- https://www.stylecraze.com/articles/simple-tips-to-look-beautiful-without-makeup/#gref
- https://www.medicalnewstoday.com/articles/14417.php#treatments
- https://isearchidealbeauty.weebly.com/conclusion-and-reflection.html
- https://www.oliebiologique.com/2012/08/31/why-go-natural-the-benefits-of-using-organic-skincare/
- https://thriveglobal.com/stories/how-to-feel-naturally-beautiful/

- https://www.philippe-naud.com/what-inorganic-skincare-products-do-to-your-body/
- https://ascc.com.au/the-benefits-of-cosmeticstoiletries/
- https://www.goodhousekeeping.com/beauty/anti-aging/tips/g2154/125-ways-to-look-young-feel-great/
- https://www.healthline.com/nutrition/13-acne-remedies#section13
- https://www.thelifeco.com/en/anti-aging/9-natural-anti-aging-secrets/
- https://www.wikihow.com/Determine-Your-Skin-Type
- https://www.teamiblends.com/blogs/lifestyle/learn-how-to-get-rid-of-blemishes-with-these-proven-tips
- https://www.wikihow.com/Get-Rid-of-Cellulite
- https://www.wikihow.com/Treat-Eczema-Naturally
- https://doctor.ndtv.com/skin/8-simple-ways-to-get-rid-of-wrinkles-on-the-face-naturally-1836103

www.ingramcontent.com/pod-product-compliance
Lightning Source LLC
Chambersburg PA
CBHW031918270726
48655CB00006BA/2709